Detox Diet: Sugar Detox:

Detox Cleanse to Heal the Inflammation, Lose Belly Fat & Increase Energy

Emma Rose

Detox Diet Guide

Lose Weight Quickly, Achieve Optimal Health and Feel Energized Through the 10 Day Detox

Emma Rose

Table of Contents

Introduction

I want to thank you and congratulate you for purchasing the book, *"Detox Diet Guide: Lose Weight Quickly, Achieve Optimal Health and Feel Energized Through the 10 Day Detox"*.

This book contains proven steps and strategies on how to not just simply flush out toxic substances from our bodies, but to also enhance the way our bodies naturally flush out those toxins.

It also contains other important information such as the most common toxins that are found in the environment that we unknowingly consume, the many ways our bodies naturally detoxify themselves, the things one must and must not do within the ten days of the detox diet, detoxification recipes that can be easily prepared, and some important reminders that must be taken before, during, and after the detox diet.

Thanks again for purchasing this book. I hope you enjoy it! Please take some time to stop by and LIKE our Facebook page:

https://www.facebook.com/joypublishing

With gratitude,

Emma Rose

Chapter 1: Toxins and the Body

As the human body does its usual processes, some things need to be expelled. These are usually waste products made as a result of filtering out substances not needed by the body. There is a reason for the so-called "calls of nature" – which are peeing and releasing excrement.

But sometimes, those unwanted substances can build up in the organs and the bodily systems that comprise them. If there are too much of those substances, they will cause all sorts of harm to the overall bodily functions that can lead to various ailments.

The Top 10 List of Most Common Toxins

Human civilization evolves as a result of the desire of the people to live more comfortably and conveniently. But in the process of that evolution, it has unknowingly unleashed a cavalcade of impurities that do not just pollute the environment, but also the human body. Despite the many efforts by several government agencies and private individuals to thwart the sources of those impurities, there are traces of those impurities that still linger around. Those traces remain in the air, in the soil, in several bodies of water – and eventually, in the foods that humanity consumes.

According to Dr. Joseph Mercola, a well-known personality in the US wellness movement and owner and founder of Mercola.com (one of the most-trusted health websites), the ten most common toxic substances that are still prevalent in the environment to this day are the following:

1. Polychlorinated biphenyls, or PCBs, were commonly dumped by factories into nearby bodies of water. Due to their toxicity, PCBs were banned decades ago. However, traces of PCBs can still be found in those bodies of water since the toxic substances do not break down easily even after all those years. Fish that swim in those bodies of water still consume PCBs unknowingly. As people still eat those fish, they will also ingest

PCBs that will contribute to ailments such as cancer and brain defects in newborn babies.

2. Pesticides, while they do kill pests as their name says, are the major contributors of cancer. As farms still use synthetic pesticides such as weed killers, fungi killers, and insect killers; residues of those pesticides still remain in as much as 50 to 90 percent of US farm produce. Furthermore, there are bug sprays used to kill cockroaches and other unwanted insects in homes. Those bug sprays also contain the same carcinogenic substances as farm-focused pesticides. Besides cancer, pesticides also cause Parkinson's disease, miscarriage, nerve damage, birth defects, and getting in the way of nutrient absorption.

3. Fungal toxins not just come in the form of poisonous mushrooms. The most common of those fungal toxins is mold. Mold thrives in moist places such as bathrooms and kitchens; and can even sustain in vulnerable foods such as peanuts, wheat, and corn. One in three people are allergic to this fungal toxin. If left unchecked, mold causes cancer, heart disease, asthma, multiple sclerosis, and diabetes.

4. Phthalates are commonly found in plastic products and are responsible for softening them, making them easier to mold. They can seep into foodstuffs and drinks that are placed inside plastic food containers and plastic bottles. The result of ingesting too much phthalates is hormonal imbalance, since the substances resemble naturally-produced hormones. In children, phthalates can stunt their growth.

5. Volatile organic compounds, or VOCs, are commonly found in several household products such as air fresheners, cleaning fluids, mothballs, and varnishes. VOCs aid in air pollution and cause several sicknesses such as cancer, irritation of eyes and lungs, headaches, dizziness, and impaired memory.

6. Dioxins are some of the pollutants that are produced when something is burned, especially in massive quantities. As they are released into the air, humans not just breathe in the dioxins. Livestock can also inhale those toxins and settle in

4

their fats even after they are brought to the slaughterhouse to be made into meat. Dioxins cause cancer, stunted growth, reproductive system impairments, skin disorders such as acne, and slight damage to the liver.

7. Asbestos was a popular insulation material, but it was banned in the seventies due to its carcinogenic effects. Traces of asbestos can still be found in old homes that did not have their insulations replaced. Besides cancer, asbestos causes scarring on the lung tissue.

8. Toxic heavy metals such as lead, arsenic, and mercury can still be found in various objects such as cheaply-made toys, preserved wood, antiperspirants, and building materials. Once those metals are inhaled or ingested, they can cause cancer, brain and nerve disorders such as Alzheimer's disease, nausea, lesser amounts of red and white blood cells, and abnormal heartbeats.

9. Chloroform is a common chemical that is used to make other chemicals. It is prevalent in the air, in water, and in food. It can cause cancer, infertility, birth defects, headaches, dizziness, and damage to the liver and kidneys.

10. Chlorine is commonly found in water as it is used to purify it. Whether from the typical drinking water or from a swimming pool, too much of chlorine will cause all sorts of respiratory problems such as sore throat, accumulation of fluid in the lungs, and asthma.

Based on this list, many of those toxins in the environment are brought about by humanity's modern lifestyles. Before they do undue harm to the body, especially the dreaded cancer, they must be flushed out promptly.

Other Sources of Toxins

Besides the ten most common toxic substances, there are also other toxins that can be found in almost everything in the modern world. It is inevitable that one must intake those toxins unknowingly, one way or the other.

The two most popular vices, which are smoking and drinking, are the other major reasons for the body's toxicity. Both alcohol and nicotine have been proven many times by the scientific community to be not just toxic, but also addicting. Those two substances also alter the brain's functions. Other toxic substances include caffeine, empty sugars, and saturated fats. The latter two are especially notorious for being fat fodder since they cannot be processed into needed energy.

Many cosmetics today also contain toxic substances such as VOCs that can be absorbed into the skin. Some cosmetics producers have already taken steps in ridding their beauty products of those toxins.

Taking too many medications all at once can also cause the body to be laced with toxins, since they are not properly eliminated from the body. If the body feels too taxed from a cornucopia of meds, a consultation with the doctor will help.

There are also naturally-occurring toxins that are used by certain plants and animals as defense mechanisms against invaders. Snakes and jellyfish have highly deadly toxins and should not be consumed as food. A Japanese dish called *fugu* uses a type of blowfish that releases toxins which will certainly kill someone who eats an improperly-prepared version of the dish.

Processed foods, especially canned goods, are also a major source of toxins. While those foods contain preservatives that prolong their shelf lives, they unknowingly unleash a world of hurt on one who voraciously eats these. Needless to say, one must balance those foods out with naturally-grown foods.

Chapter 2: Why Must We Detoxify?

Detoxification is not just the simple flushing out of unwanted substances when the body cannot handle expelling them on its own. It is also the purging of impure thoughts in the mind that cause all sorts of decisions to inhale and ingest several toxins, whether knowingly or unknowingly, into the body. To ensure that an individual is rightfully clean in both body and mind, all sorts of unwanted things must be eliminated, especially in the detox diet.

The Body Does It Own Job...

The excretory system does its job of purging waste substances from the body via its two major processes: urination and release of excrement. Urination is obviously handled by the urinary system, while the release of excrement is handled by the lower parts of the digestive system.

The urinary system's main actor is the kidneys. The kidneys filter unwanted stuff such as ammonia, urea, uric acid, and excess salt and water from the blood as well as other bodily fluids. Those unwanted stuff then get to the bladder, which acts as a temporary storage. If the bladder gets full, the stuff gets expelled out of the urethra in the form of urine. Ammonia is a byproduct of the breakdown and usage of protein for the body's energy, while urea and uric acid are less toxic substances that result from the breakdown of ammonia.

The lower parts of the digestive system consist of the liver, the intestines, and the colon. The liver does its job of breaking down foreign substances so that the kidneys can have an easier job filtering them out as urine. The intestines and the colon facilitate the expelling of solid waste substances in the form of feces. The colon, in particular, absorbs trace minerals such as potassium and sends them to the bloodstream before they are included as feces that will be expelled by pooping.

Another natural detoxifier found in the human body is the lymphatic system. The lymphatic system contains lymph nodes that are scattered throughout the body but are interconnected. Those nodes provide the body with immunity, complementing the immune system, by filtering out unwelcome invaders such as bacteria, viruses, old red blood cells, and other toxic substances.

Other parts of the excretory system consist of the lungs and skin. The lungs expel excess water and carbon dioxide when someone breathes out. The skin kicks out excess water, salt, uric acid, and excess trace minerals in the form of sweat.

...But It Is Not Enough in the Modern Age

However, as demonstrated in the previous chapter, there are far too many substances that are deemed toxic in the wrong amounts. With humanity's modern lifestyles, the body does not know what to make of the increasing number of unwelcome invaders in its insides. These usually never get flushed out as urine and feces, but instead accumulate in the body fat.

As the invaders multiply and never get flushed out, they get in the way of the body's usual processes and will cause several problems such as depleted energy levels, unnatural weight gain, and various diseases that target the major body systems.

Another thing that is not helping the body in its natural detoxification process is the busy and hectic schedules people normally have. Because those people have no time to perform even mundane healthy tasks such as drinking adequate water, the body never gets its supply of natural detox assistants. Couple the lack of those assistants with stress and it will be a recipe for disaster.

Therefore, it is important that in this world of toxicity, people must amplify their bodily defenses against all sorts of foreign toxic substances by enhancing the many components of the excretory system such as the kidneys, the liver, the intestines, and the colon. With the contaminants out of the way, the body's natural healing processes also get their groove back. As the major organ systems work hand-in-hand, the benefits that are felt in one particular system will spread towards the other systems.

In short, steeling the body and its functions, especially the excretory functions, is one of the first lines of defense against toxin-induced sicknesses. There will be a marked loss in weight, since the excessive fats as well as the toxins they contain are properly expelled. There will also be renewed liveliness since the bodily functions that have something to do with the intake and processing of energy sources are no longer clogged by invasive toxins.

Why the Mind Is Also Important in Detoxification

The decisions a person makes, no matter how small they are, can contribute to huge consequences. For example, if one decides to commute to a bar, he or she gets all sorts of toxins in the process – airborne impurities from urban roads, food additives from the snacks he or she eats while commuting, nicotine and other chemicals from tobacco smoke generated by smokers inside and outside the bar, and alcohol from the hard drinks he or she consumes while in the bar.

Therefore, it is important that a person must think thoroughly and deeply before settling on a decision that will make him or her take in all those unwanted toxins along the way. Yes, this may turn him or her into a control freak, but there are also decisions that will endow him or her with long-term benefits. Remember, detoxification starts in the mind. The decisions that lead to the unknowing intake of toxins must be sorted out and eliminated from the usual routines first.

Chapter 3: The Crucial Ten Days

There are several forms of detoxification, and they more often than not involve ingesting special liquids and solids, cleansing the colon, foot baths and foot pads, spas and saunas, and fasting. But they also cost money, are always focused on the short-term effects, and may not deliver the detoxification results one desires. The best form of the detox diet must involve getting rid of major sources of toxins, ingesting more of the substances that will greatly assist the body's natural detoxification processes, never integrating any form of starvation or elimination of a major food group from the diet, and clearing the mind of impure thoughts that lead to impure actions. This way, the diet will grant long-term effects of well-being. As a beneficial consequence, this diet will cost little to no money, except for the money to be spent on detoxifying foods and drinks.

The ten days this detox diet contains are important to ensure natural weight loss and general well-being. And even after the diet period ends, some good habits contained in this diet, particularly the continued eating of healthy foods, must still be kept. This is to ensure that the person undergoing this diet will transition into a healthy lifestyle.

Preparing for the Diet

One important thing to do when undergoing this diet, or any other diet for that matter, is to not rush in immediately. A crash diet will have nasty consequences such as abrupt changing of body patterns that lead to all sorts of ailments as well as retention of the weight one lost during the diet routine. Therefore, one must start slow and transition into the diet carefully.

Not rushing in also applies to the chewing of food. The body needs some time to digest the food. Never treat the ten days of the diet like some kind of work deadline.

The usual vice-based sources of toxins, which are tobacco and alcohol, must be eliminated first. While dealing with the withdrawal effects of both of those substances may be difficult, timely help from a doctor who has a specialization in several types of addictions and substance abuse will lessen the difficulty.

In the three days before the actual start of the diet, rid the pantry and fridge of tempting foodstuffs that are loaded with empty calories. These include sweets and most forms of processed foods and fast food. At the same time, steadily increase the intake of fruits and vegetables – *especially organic ones.* As much as possible, turn the veggies into freshly-prepared salads and/or lightly steam them. As for the fruits, eat them raw and/or turn them into natural juices.

Since pesticide residue in fruits and vegetables is inevitable, the use of fruit and vegetable washes must be prioritized.

The intake of caffeine must be slowly and surely reduced to prevent withdrawal symptoms such as headaches. Switching to decaf coffee and low-caffeine teas such as green tea will help, as is the trick of diluting regular coffee and tea in huge amounts of water.

And speaking of water, the time-tested advice of eight to ten glasses of water a day will especially help the detox diet become successful. Drink it throughout the ten days of the diet.

Aromatherapy using essential oils is helpful, as this therapy helps to calm the mind in order for it to prepare for the rigors of the critical ten days.

Finally, before embarking on the detox diet itself, please consult a registered dietician who can recommend the detoxifying foods to be eaten based on your genetic makeup. Furthermore, *do not stop* taking prescribed medicine, as discontinuing medications can have devastating effects on the body. Diets are not meant to be one-man shows, especially if the individual still has to learn much about the intricacies of diet programs like this.

Eat and Drink Them

With the transition phase over, it is time to actually start the detox diet. Here is a comprehensive list of foods and drinks that must be ingested during the ten crucial days of the diet.

1. Organic fruits and vegetables are the main focus of the detox diet. It does not matter what the size or type of fruit or vegetable one will be consuming – as long as it is free of pesticides and synthetic fertilizers and is grown using age-old farming techniques, it certainly counts. Eat a good variety of fruits and vegetables to round out all the necessary nutrients.

2. Brown rice is much healthier compared to the typical white rice. As white rice is a result of the milling process, brown rice retains some nutrients that are usually lost during milling. This type of rice is also a rich source of fiber, which will aid in flushing the toxins out via the intestines and the colon.

3. Herbs are permissible, since they are also plants. Use them to flavor the dishes as well as utilize them for aromatherapy. Herbal teas are also a-OK, since they do not contain caffeine at all. As with fruits and vegetables, herbs must not have traces of anything toxic.

4. Whole-grain products, much like brown rice, do not undergo the nutrient-losing milling process. They are also rich sources of fiber. Whole-grain products include whole wheat bread, bran, and rolled oats.

5. Seaweeds such as kelp and *nori* wrappers used for sushi are also plant-based. They can also be consumed the same way as typical veggies do.

6. Beans such as green peas, chick peas, lentils, kidney beans, and black beans are permitted.

7. One can go nuts with nuts and seeds. Allowable things include almonds, cashews, walnuts, watermelon seeds, pumpkin seeds, sunflower seeds, and sesame seeds. As a general rule, pick only raw, unsalted nuts and seeds.

8. Coconuts, while they are not actually nuts, are also allowed. There are several coconut-based consumables such as coconut water and coconut oil. One can also eat fresh coconut meat straight from the source.

9. Plant-based oils are encouraged. Olive oil, especially the extra virgin kind, is highly recommended.

10. Round out the protein-based nutrition with plant-based protein sources such as soy. Soy milk and tofu are easily-acquired sources of plant-based protein.

11. All sorts of edible mushrooms are permitted. Portobello and shiitake mushrooms can act as good substitutes for meat.

12. Natural sweeteners such as raw honey and natural maple syrup are permitted.

13. Besides herbs, other natural condiments that are tolerable include apple cider vinegar, sea salt, and mustard.

14. If there is still a desire to eat meat and get adequate protein, go with lean meats such as fish and organic chicken. Eggs are also on the list, as long as they are organic.

Never Eat and Drink Them

Meanwhile, these are the foods and drinks to avoid during the detox diet phase.

1. In general, non-lean types of red meat are off-limits. Canned meat is especially forbidden.

2. All forms of processed foods containing all sorts of additives and preservatives are out of the question. On a related note, artificial sweeteners and processed condiments are also out.

3. Typical white sugar and brown sugar are verboten, as well as high-fructose syrups.

4. Corn must be avoided as it is acid-forming. The acid in question is uric acid. Furthermore, the corn kernels that are indigestible will make bathroom breaks more excruciating.

5. While nuts are OK, peanuts and peanut butter are usually excluded.

6. Milk is normally not allowed, but half a cup of yogurt containing good bacteria per day is an exception to that.

7. Caffeine is another typical forbidden substance.

8. Shortening and margarine are inadmissible.

9. While fish is OK, other seafoods are not.

Other Cleansing Procedures

There are many variations of the detox diet, but the one being presented in this book will not involve complicated doohickeys and specialized food and drinks to amplify the detoxification effect. Here are some things one can also do during the ten days of the diet.

With all the conveniences of Internet-based connectivity, sometimes too much is too much. Dedicate one of the ten days, or even all ten days, to a temporary break from technology. Put away the smartphone or tablet, avoid touching the computer, and never be tempted to go online just about anywhere. Take the time off from technology to visit someplace serene, like a retreat house. This technology break will clear the mind of all sorts of burdening thoughts that may poison one's thinking the same way that bodily toxins do.

Take some time off to scrape the tongue. Tongue scraping is a practice in ayurvedic medicine, or ancient Hindu medicine, where all the impurities built up on the tongue are removed. Tongue scrapers can be bought for cheap at drug store.

Try to write all the stored thoughts and feelings, even negative ones, into a diary or notebook. Releasing all the stored strong emotions to a diary or notebook has a cathartic effect, since keeping those emotions locked away will eventually take the toll on one's health.

Another mind-cleansing procedure one can do during the ten days is meditation. Meditation also helps clear the mind of toxic thoughts that lead to stress, which then slows down the liver's detoxification process. Yoga is especially helpful as a meditation tool. You may also augment your meditation by doing deep breathing exercises or visualizing relaxing images such as watching the sunset at the beach.

Get enough dosages of vitamin C. While the vitamin is better known for boosting immunity, it also helps the body with the production of glutathione. Glutathione may be better known as a skin rejuvenating agent, but it also exists in the liver as a detoxification aid. Citrus fruits are the best-known sources of vitamin C.

Enhance blood circulation, since poor blood circulation will hamper the flushing out of impurities from the blood. Exercise is a guaranteed way to get that blood pumping.

Keep in mind that not all bacteria are bad. Good bacteria mostly reside in the intestines, aiding in digestion and preventing bad bacteria from releasing toxins that can be deployed in the bloodstream. Help the good bacteria by taking probiotic drinks.

Chapter 4: Detoxification Recipes

Breakfast Recipes

Gut-Busting Oatmeal Bowl

Ingredients:

- 1-2 cups oatmeal

- 1-2 cups water or nut milk

- A mixture of fresh berries and fresh fruits, all sliced

Procedure:

1. Prepare the oatmeal as indicated in the packaging.

2. While hot, pour the berries and fruits onto the prepared oatmeal, and mix.

Berry Blast Smoothie

Ingredients:

- 1-2 cups mixed fresh berries
- 1-2 cups protein powder
- 1-2 cups ice cubes

Procedure:

1. Throw all the ingredients into a blender, and hit puree.
2. Serve the smoothie in a tall glass.

Lunch Recipes

Veggie Cavalcade Salad with Tofu

Ingredients:

- 6-8 pieces of any whole vegetable (for greens, an amount of at least five leaves equals one whole piece)

- 1-2 pieces tofu, diced

- 4-5 teaspoons extra virgin olive oil

- 2 teaspoons fresh lemon juice

- 1 teaspoon freshly-chopped herbs of choice

Procedure:

1. Fry the tofu in 2-3 teaspoons olive oil until slightly browned. Set aside.

2. Slice and/or dice the vegetables into reasonably-sized pieces. Leave the greens untouched.

3. Pour all the vegetables and the tofu into a bowl. Mix completely.

4. Combine 2 teaspoons olive oil, the lemon juice, and the herbs to make the dressing.

5. Pour the dressing all over the salad. Mix completely.

Special Omelet Rice

Ingredients:

- 3-5 organic eggs

- Fresh or dried herbs (any variety), to taste

- 2-3 teaspoons extra virgin olive oil

- 1-2 cups cooked brown rice

Procedure:

1. Beat the eggs into a scramble while adding the herbs.

2. Pour the olive oil into a heated pan. Wait until the oil is hot.

3. Pour the egg and herb mixture until the omelet is formed. Turn over to ensure proper cooking.

4. Once the omelet is out of the pan, place the brown rice inside it. Make sure the omelet wraps around the rice.

5. Serve hot with mustard.

Dinner Recipes

<u>The Steamed Medley</u>

Ingredients:

- 1 slice salmon
- 5-10 pieces broccoli and asparagus (can be of any combination)
- 1/4 cup fresh lemon juice
- Fresh or dried herbs (any variety), to taste

Procedure:

1. In a steamer or a rice cooker with a steaming basket, arrange the salmon slice and the broccoli and asparagus pieces so that the steam will be evenly distributed.

2. Sprinkle the salmon and the vegetables with the lemon juice and fresh herbs.

3. Begin steaming the salmon and the vegetables. Seven to ten minutes is enough for the lemon and the herbs to seep into the steamed content.

4. Serve hot.

Glorified Bunch of Small Potatoes

Ingredients:

- 6 ounces small potatoes
- 4 tablespoons extra virgin olive oil
- Any natural condiment of choice

Procedure:

1. Gently simmer the potatoes in water for 5-10 minutes. Drain them off afterwards. Retain the peels beforehand.

2. Heat the olive oil in a roasting tin, but not to burning levels.

3. Roast every side of the potatoes until crisp and golden brown. This will take at most 45 minutes.

4. Serve hot with the condiment of choice.

Snack and Drink Recipes

<u>Veggie Brown Rice Sushi</u>

Ingredients:

- 1 cup cooked brown rice

- 1 *nori* wrapper

- Any sliced or diced vegetable that can fit inside the sushi

Procedure:

1. Mold the brown rice into any shape, whether in a tube form or rolled into a ball. The important thing is that the vegetable must fit inside the sushi.

2. Wrap the *nori* wrapper around the formed brown rice.

3. Repeat steps 1 and 2 for any remaining amounts of vegetables, brown rice, and the *nori* wrapper.

Stretched Herbal Iced Tea

Ingredients:

- 1 bag herbal tea (any kind)
- 1 citrus fruit of choice (e.g. lemon or orange)
- 1 cup briskly-boiled water
- 2-3 cups lukewarm water
- Several ice cubes
- Honey, to taste

Procedure:

1. Depending on the strength of the resultant tea, submerge one teabag into briskly-boiled water.

2. Meanwhile, cut the citrus fruit of choice into slices that can be fit inside a glass.

3. Place the fruit slices into a tall glass that can accommodate at least five cups.

4. Carefully pour both the brewed tea and the lukewarm water into the tall glass at a distance of at least 12 inches from the glass. This is where the "stretched" part comes from, and one must avoid spills during the stretching process.

5. Add some dollops of honey based on the preferred amount of sweetness.

6. Finally, add the ice cubes.

Fruity Shaved Ice

Ingredients:

- 1-2 cups shaved ice

- 1/2-1 cup natural unsweetened fruit juice of any kind

Procedure:

1. Place the shaved ice in either a wide glass or a bowl.

2. Pour the unsweetened fruit juice on top of the shaved ice, and enjoy.

Note: One can replace shaved ice with shaved or crushed frozen fruit.

Chapter 5: Some Friendly Reminders

As with every other diet program on the planet, care, precise planning, patience, and perseverance must be taken to heart when undergoing the detoxification diet. Even in a short period like ten days, many things will happen. To ensure that the detox diet will become a success that will beget many more successes in the realm of the healthy lifestyle, keep the following friendly reminders in mind.

Do Not Starve

Other detox diets recommend taking only the formulas they sell themselves. Indeed, they may contain needed plant-based nourishment needed for detoxification, but the makers of those diets often forget that an imbalanced diet that is lacking in calories will prove detrimental to the body. Not only will the energy levels be depleted, but the metabolism process will also be slowed down. One unpleasant aftereffect is the tendency to eat more, especially unhealthy foods, once the diet period is over. This will make natural weight loss almost unachievable. Even worse, the lack of micronutrients in these other detox diets will lead to malnutrition that is based on micronutrient deficiency, which opens yet another floodgate of diseases. Other nasty effects of other detox crash diets include muscle degeneration, since the muscles have no source of energy to turn to, and an imbalance in blood sugar levels.

Hence, this detox diet espouses the idea that *forced starvation is absolutely prohibited.* Just eat the recommended foods at will and in good, moderated amounts.

Expect to Pee (and Poop and Sweat) a Lot

Since the detox diet enhances the body's natural detox functions, expect one undergoing the diet to pee a lot. Water, in particular, helps in flushing out toxins.

Excessive peeing not just happens when the detox diet goes overboard. Excessive sweating also happens, as well as the resultant excrement being too liquid and nasty-smelling. Peeing, pooping, and sweating too much can lead to dehydration if the amount of fluids being taken is not immediately replenished.

Dehydration is not just the depletion of the body's water, but is also the disrupted balance of fluids and electrolytes that can lead to ailments such as gastrointestinal distress, headaches, fatigue, irritability, skin irritations, circulatory problems, kidney failure, and heat stroke. Death also awaits one who is severely dehydrated.

To counteract dehydration, do not depend on fluids and fluids alone, unlike what some detox diets emphasize. Be well-balanced in both solids and liquids to avoid lost hours as a result of abnormally frequent trips to the bathroom.

Want a Colonic? No Thanks

Another form of the detox therapy involves cleansing the colon and intestines of toxins that may be released into the bloodstream. However, as demonstrated in the third chapter, there are beneficial bacteria that reside in the colon and intestines. If those bacteria are flushed out, the normal digestive process will be hampered, and the bad bacteria will have a good time releasing more toxins since their rivals are gone. The flushing out of good bacteria also results from the detox diet going beyond the recommended ten days.

Another bad effect of colon cleansing is dehydration, for the same reasons demonstrated in the previous section. Trace minerals such as potassium are also lost during the cleansing process, which contributes to dehydration. Other side effects of colon cleansing include nausea and vomiting.

Diet as an End to the Means, Not a Means to the End

People who want the figures of their dreams often forget that dieting is not really meant to immediately shed unwanted pounds.

Dieting is truly meant for improved nourishment and nutrition. The notions of shedding that slab or beer belly in preparation for an event like showing off in a bikini should be disposed of. A proper mindset must be established first when doing the detox diet or any other diet for that matter.

As stated before, the detox diet being demonstrated in this book should be a transitional phase to a healthier lifestyle. Thinking in the long term when dieting is certainly better than thinking in the short term. One should remember that dieting must be an end to unhealthy habits and not a means to end that "awful" figure.

Conclusion

Thank you again for purchasing *"Detox Diet Guide: Lose Weight Quickly, Achieve Optimal Health and Feel Energized Through the 10 Day Detox"*!

I hope this book was able to help you to understand the ins and outs of the detox diet and why it is important to achieve a major change in only a short time.

Are you ready for the change? Tony Robbins says in order to create effective change, you need to start by being disgusted with where you are at. Are you disgusted with your health or body? Is it an ABSOLUTE MUST to change...not another moment? You need to feel the pain of where you are at to get the urgency to change and manifest the momentum to take action.

The next step is to consult your doctor or dietician before embarking on such a diet. And once you are given the final OK, you can then consult various more detoxification recipes based on the comprehensive list of allowable foods and drinks in this book. The recipes given in this book is just a starting point.

Finally, if you enjoyed this book, please take the time to share your thoughts and post a review on Amazon. It would be greatly appreciated!

I would love for you to share your experiences, stories and encouragements with me. My email address is

emmarosekindle@gmail.com

In addition, please remember to check out our Facebook page in order to find other resources and upcoming promotions:

https://www.facebook.com/joypublishing

With sincere thanks,

Emma Rose

Preview Of "Paleo Free Diet Guide for Beginners: Over 50 Paleo Free Diet Recipes for Fast Weight Loss and Optimal Health"

Introduction

I want to thank you and congratulate you for purchasing the book, *"Paleo Free Diet Guide for Beginners: Over 50 Paleo Free Diet Recipes for Optimal Health and Fast Weight Loss"*.

This book contains everything you might need to know when it comes to getting started with the Paleo diet. It is provided in an easily digestible format that allows you to better absorb the information. There are no complicated explanations about how it works! You'll be given what you need straight up so you won't have to waste time trying to understand exactly what the diet is. Whether it's for your overall good health or to lose a few pounds, Paleo can certainly help you with it. To help you get started, we'll do the same and start you off with 50 of the best Paleo recipes that you can slowly but surely shift your everyday menu to.

It's never easy changing a diet. I often fall into self pity when I can no longer have the foods I enjoy. Either I feel sorry for myself or I get rebellious and binge and anything and everything. I always knew the value of eating healthy. I could just never bring myself to do it. It wasn't until I had a miscarriage that I got serious about my health. I have made drastic changes that others just don't understand. But the pay off is the weight I've lost and the better health I'm experiencing.

My hope for you is not to be on another "diet." This isn't a restriction diet like Atkins. The goal is to have a lifestyle change. Lifestyle changes are more sustainable and maintain weight loss long term compared to restriction diets. The change is hard to start but worth it when you commit. The trick is to get the momentum to start.

Thanks again for purchasing this book. I hope you enjoy reading it and eating the recipes from it!

With gratitude,

Emma Rose

Chapter 1 – What Is the Paleo Diet?

The Paleo Diet is known by many names such as the cavemen diet, stone age diet and hunter-gatherer diet, to name a few. The concept behind this diet follows that of the Paleolithic era before the development of agriculture. Essentially, you consume the same foods that the cavemen used to eat. The focus is on eating food closest to its natural, unprocessed state. The cavemen would gather their food from any source available whether it was wild animals, berries, vegetables, or fruits. As a result, they were strong, fit, and healthy for thousands of years.

This type of diet is still very young, less than fifty years only, but more in depth researches and studies are being conducted to increase the information and knowledge on this diet. The results of previous studies conducted on the Paleo diet reveal the improvement of health to the people involved. This is attributed to the fact that no processed foods and additives are included. The Paleo Diet is a diet that works with our genetics – before machinery and processing got involved. Foods that were not available during the Paleolithic time such as dairy products, salt, sugar and grains are not included in the preparation of the Paleo diet.

The modern diet predominately consumed in the Western world is full of refined foods, trans fats, salt and sugar. These ingredients are known to indirectly cause diseases such as hypertension, diabetes, strokes, obesity and other heart problems. The list goes on even further with the increase diagnosis of cancer, Parkinson's, Alzheimer's, depression and infertility. "What an extraordinary achievement for a civilization: to have developed the one diet that reliably makes its people sick!" (Michael Pollen, Food Rules: An Eater's Manual, Penguin Books 2009).

Foods included in the Paleo Diet

- Fruit

- Vegetables

- Lean Meat

- Seafood

- Nuts/Seeds

- Healthy Fats (eg. coconut, avocado, nuts and seeds, olive oil, grass fed butter)

Foods NOT included in the Paleo Diet

- Dairy

- Grain

- Processed Food

Why not grain?

You may be surprised to see that grains are not included in the Paleo Diet. We are accustomed to grains being a part of a balanced diet. However, our bodies are not designed to deal with the nutritional components of grains such as gluten, lectin, and phytates.

Gluten is a protein substance found in wheat, barley and rye. Many people are discovering that their bodies are gluten sensitive and are eliminating gluten from their diet. The most extreme case of gluten sensitivity is Celiac Disease. Individuals with this disease can pick up the minutest trace of gluten and react immediately.

Lectin binds to insulin receptors and can also cause leptin resistance.

Phytates cause minerals to become unavailable during digestion.

Why is dairy a problem?

When purchasing milk, you need to be mindful of the source.

Check out the rest of "Paleo Diet Guide for Beginners: Over 50 Paleo Diet Recipes for Fast Weight Loss and Optimal Health" on Amazon.

Or go to: http://amzn.to/1jIJUFX

Sugar Detox Guide for Beginners

Lose Weight Quickly, Achieve Optimal Health, Feel Energized and Eliminate Sugar Cravings Naturally

Emma Rose

Table of Contents

Introduction

I want to thank you and congratulate you for purchasing the book, *"**Sugar Detox Guide for Beginners**: Lose Weight Quickly, Achieve Optimal Health, Feel Energized and Eliminate Sugar Cravings Naturally"*.

This book contains proven steps and strategies on how to detoxify your body and kick Sugar Addiction in the butt within 21 days.

Because of the way food is processed nowadays, most people don't know that almost everything they eat has lots of sugar in it. And with sugar being discovered as the real cause of obesity, heart disease and other illnesses, this is a very bad thing.

Understand Sugar Addiction, its symptoms and the detrimental health effects it has. Know exactly what sugar does to your brain and body. And most importantly, know how exactly you can kick your sugar addiction goodbye!

All my life I've had a sweet tooth. I would even go as far as to say that I had a sugar addiction! Over the last few years my sugar addiction got worse: I had dessert multiple times a day and every day (I guess being a Foods teacher didn't help much). I would joke with people by telling them that I had my servings of vegetables for the day in chocolate...except, I still didn't have the vegetables. It got pretty bad. I knew I hated eating that much dessert but I couldn't stop. I would eat one Ferrero Rocher and then go back for another. As I walked back to the treats, I would pass the mirror and think to myself, "I don't need to have this chocolate. But, ah, what the heck, I don't care." In the end, I'd have about 6 Ferrero Rochers in addition to the other treats I had earlier that day.

Finally, I had to take the huge tray of Ferrero Rochers to school to give to my students on Valentine's Day. There was no way I could eat the other 30 myself. Eating all this sugar caused a huge war within me. I knew that my extreme sugar eating was unhealthy for me but I didn't want to stop. I loved it too much. As a result, I wrestled between the ideal of where I wanted to be and the reality of where I was. I knew I had the discipline to say no to other things, so why couldn't I say no to chocolate?

I eventually came to the point where I was starting to get fed up with not feeling well. I had a lot of chronic pain in my neck and I was constantly tired. I knew that sugar was irritating the problem and causing inflammation in my body. At was starting to reach the breaking point. Ultimately, I chose to go off of sugar for at least three weeks to break the habit I had created for myself. It was seriously a miracle to stay consistent with my goal because I really didn't want to give up my favorite desserts.

I encourage you to make that switch to healthier and happier lifestyle. Cutting out all the processed foods and going back to the basics really does clear up the body and help it function better. I've seen the changes in my own life as hard as it's been to make those changes. You, too, can make the changes necessary and still have your sweets along the way!

Thanks again for purchasing this book, I hope you enjoy it! Please take some time to stop by and LIKE our Facebook page:

https://www.facebook.com/joypublishing

With gratitude,

Emma Rose

Chapter 1

The Problem with Too Much Sugar...

For years, nutritionist have pinned all the caution warning on fats and other additives found in everyone's diets. But the real cause of all the obesity and other complications have been uncovered from the role it plays to weaken your diet and your body.

- *Sugar has no essential nutrients and spells trouble for your teeth.*

  A lot of sugar additives have high levels of calories with literally no essential nutrients, which is why they are called the Empty Calories. When it is said that there are no essential nutrients, it means no proteins, fats, vitamins or minerals, all that is in sugar is just pure energy. If the amount of sugar in your calorie intake goes up to 10 or 20 percent, you'll start having problems in nutrient deficiencies and more.

  Also, being a substance of easily convertible energy, it means that it is not only your body that gets a boost, so does the bad bacteria in your mouth. That could be a major disaster for your teeth. It feeds the bacteria so they multiply faster, harming your mouth (and body) faster.

- *Fructose can overload your liver.*

Sugar is broken down into two simple sugar compounds before it enters the bloodstream. These are fructose and glucose. Glucose can be found in every living cell in all organisms. If you don't consume enough of it from your foods, your body would provide it for you. Now the problematic one is fructose. It is not naturally occurring in your body so you can only get it through your diet. Your body does not really need fructose in order to function properly, but it does taste good.

Fructose is not inherently bad because we do get it from eating fruits, but the only organ that can metabolize it properly is the liver, and it stores the processed fructose as glycogen until your body needs it. Now, if the liver is already full of glycogen, it will transform the rest of the fructose (if you keep on digesting too much) into fat. And this can turn into a fatty-liver problem.

This is usually not a problem who are physically active. Healthy, active people metabolize their fructose faster before it can become a burden to their bodies. This is compared to people who have a sedentary lifestyle who ingest the same high-calorie, high-sugar diet.

- *Sugar can cause insulin resistance that can drive towards diabetes.*

We know that insulin helps the cells focus on burning glucose instead of fat when blood sugar enters these cells. Insulin resistance is caused by the insulin hormone stopping from working properly. Too much glucose in the blood is very toxic and causes the complications of diabetes, like going blind.

When the cells become resistant to insulin, the glucose stacks up in them and contributes to the onset of diseases. These may include obesity, metabolic syndrome, cardiovascular diseases and most commonly, diabetes (type II). Large amounts of sugar consumed have always been associated with insulin resistance.

- *Sugar has fat-promoting effects.*

  Different food types have different effects on the brain and hormones, particularly those that deal with controlling the appetite. Glucose and fructose have opposite effects on the satiation of hunger.

  In a certain medical study, those who drank fructose-sweetened beverages actually become hungrier while those sweetened with glucose got lowered levels of the hunger hormone, Ghrelin. Sugar can provide energy, but it cannot remove hunger, thus this contributes to an increase in calorie intake.

- *Sugar is highly addictive.*

  Sugar causes massive releases of dopamine in the brain. This is like your brain rewarding the body for something it likes. Because of this, people susceptible to addiction become hooked to sugary foods as well as junk foods.

  The problem in the saying "Everything in Moderation" is it does not work for people addicted to sugar. The only thing that will help with this true addiction is to completely remove sugars from your diet.

- *It's the sugar and not the fat that raises the cholesterol and contributes to heart disease.*

The world has always blamed saturated fats for heart diseases, which by the way, is the leading cause of death in the world. But, newer studies show that it is not fat but fructose that causes harm to the body's metabolism and thus contribute to diseases. That does not mean that fructose is inherently bad, only that the massive doses of fructose takes a toll on the body over time. After all, fructose is used in just about everything nowadays, especially sweetened beverages and processed food.

It has been proven that stacking up sugar in the blood and cells can raise the small, dense LDL and oxidized LDL triglycerides (also known as very bad stuff!) within mere weeks. And at the same time, the built up fructose also raise blood sugar, insulin levels and abdominal obesity. And this all spell risks for heart diseases.

Chapter 2

How Do You Know You're Addicted to Sugar?

Addiction to sugar is associated to a persistent imbalance in the blood sugar, letting the body show signs and symptoms for the condition. Here are a few observed behavioral and physiological signs that you've become addicted to sugar:

- You have a craving for bread products, sugary beverages, or sweets. This is the most common and easily discernible symptom, so keep watch.

- You have what they call the food coma. It is the feeling of drowsiness and fatigue after a heavy meal. It has always been attributed to eating too much, but now we know that this is the body trying to deal with the sugar influx.

- When you miss a meal, you get a feeling of lightheadedness. Sometimes, you might even feel faint and dizzy, with the accompanying sense of irritation because of bright lights (or even just regular light). If your body gets used to a high energy, high calorie intake every time, missing a meal can make your body go into withdrawal.

- When, after you eat some sweets you get a craving for more. Actually, you feel the craving more once you've eaten the sweets. This is because the fructose in the sugar, by encouraging production of ghrelin, increases the feeling of hunger. This makes for a good appetizer and a bad snack.

- You have become dependent on caffeine to get your body started. You keep looking for coffee and sodas in order to stay awake and keep going.

- You have hard time losing weight; more so than average people. This is not because of your genes and definitely not from being too fat. This is your body being too busy dealing with all that sugar to actually start burning fat.

Usually, these can be alleviated or even completely removed by balancing your blood sugar. Here are the tried and tested methods to do just that:

- Eat more proteins. Protein promotes muscle-building which can help to metabolize your excess fats. For this, you have to ensure that you are digesting them properly. You can check this by monitoring the levels of your stomach acids.

- Eliminate sugar and carbohydrates from your diet. They are good for instant energy but bad for your sugar addiction. Eating regular, healthy meals regularly should be sufficient for your energy needs.

- Eat more good fats, complex carbohydrates, fiber and essential nutrients. A craving for sugar can come from your body not getting enough nutrients. Fiber-rich foods are also great for detoxifying your body not only from the build-up of sugar, but also from fats and other toxins.

- Detoxify your body from sugar!

It may prove to be a challenge at first, but doing the detox will definitely fix your blood sugar imbalance. And it will set up the stage for an opportunity to fix all other flaws in your diet.

It is reported that sugar addiction is even worse than other kinds of addiction. You might find that it is more difficult to get over, since there is sugar in almost everything you eat and drink, but once you have decided, and you successfully keep at it for these three weeks, you'll see results that you will be proud of.

Chapter 3

Why? How Do You Get Addicted?

It is estimated that sugar is around eight times more addictive than cocaine. Most people would have you think that sugar addiction is just a psychological eating disorder, or that it is just caused by your emotional state. That is not the case. It is a biological addiction, a disorder of the hormones and an error in the chemical balance in your body that causes cravings for sugars and carbohydrates. This will lead to uncontrollable binge eating. There has been a recent study showing that a high-sugar drink has the same addictive effect to the brain as a food-product spiked with cocaine or even morphine.

Most people would not notice that they have a full-blown sugar addiction. This is because they don't know that sugar is in everything that they eat. There was even an event where nutritionists requested food manufacturers to decrease the amount of sugar incorporated into their processed food by 30% to stop an incoming wave of diseases. Nobody reacted to the announcement because the idea was deemed absurd. What? There is sugar in a can of tomato soup? Actually, there is at least four teaspoons of sugar in each serving of that stuff.

When digesting sugar, your brain releases a kind of hormone that gives a wave of good feeling. And at the same time, that feeling activates the addiction center in the brain. Your body, liking the reaction from the stuff, will make you want more and more of it. Since sugar can be found in most food items available, you'll end up overeating, risking ingesting too much of both sugar and carbohydrates than what can be good for your body.

By developing a habit of having a constant high level of sugar in your blood, your body slowly gets used to this diet. Once you miss a meal or when you try to lower your blood sugar, your body then rejects the change. This is what happens when you experience "sugar withdrawal". Many would just use this excuse to eat more sugary sweets. But you have to see that it will only feel horrible at first. Slowly getting your diet back on the right track is worth the trouble.

Chapter 4

How Do Detox Works? Why Detox?

The detoxification works by over-correcting your body's sugar balance. This is done by completely removing sugars from your diet for a period of time to clear out any of the excess sugars before letting you return to your regular (not the sugary-regular, just regular) diet. This process can make you experience some effect that people call "Sugar Withdrawal Syndrome" that may last from a few days to a week. Mostly, it would be better to just muster up all your will power to get over these symptoms, since it will fade as you go along with the detox program. For those experiencing especially serious withdrawal symptoms, physical activity and drinking a lot of water every day will help a lot to ease the conditions. This will also include drinking water when you do feel the huge waves of food/sugar cravings that will attack you through the entire process.

So if the withdrawal can get unpleasant, why detox? Firstly, feeling worse about it actually means you are really getting better and that your body is getting rid of the built up sugar in your blood. Most of all, there are more benefits to sugar detox than just decreasing or removing your excessive craving for sweets. Some of these pluses are:

- You will begin to lose fat faster and easier. You might even find that your body's fat has gone down during the detox.

- You will feel less bloated. It is a feeling attributed to the time during or after a meal. Sugar imbalance also gives the bloated feeling that can persist throughout the day.

- Your tastes will return to normal. That would mean that healthier food will taste better since your sense is not tuned to preferring sweetness anymore. It is like removing your taste buds' bias towards sweet things. You'll be able to enjoy different kinds of food more.

- Your skin will appear clearer. Sugary diets zap out the collagen in your skin, making your complexion look blotchy and pallid. After detox, since you've lessened the sugar and increased water intake, you'll find that your skin has become better-looking than ever.

- You'll have more control over your hunger. After the detox process, you will see that you no longer have random attacks of cravings for sugar, or other food, for that matter.

- You'll have more energy and you'll feel it consistently throughout your day. There will be no more noon times after lunch spent being drowsy.

- You will have a more regular bowel movement. This is seen in detox diets that focus on removing excess sugar and carbs, promoting fiber and other essential nutrients in the process.

- Your attitude might improve, with less depressed moments and a general elevation of mood. Although this mostly comes from the knowledge that you are doing what is good for your body.

- You will definitely lower your body cholesterol; in fact, it would be great to combine this sugar detox program with physical exercise.

- You'll sleep better. A healthy diet usually helps create better sleeping habits.

Other than these physical and behavioral improvements, this sugar detox will also let you have a happier and healthier outlook on life that will help you set up the stage for creating the lifestyle that you have always wanted. Create a goal of making a lifestyle that will let you live longer, healthier, and happier!

Chapter 5

How to Start Detox?

There are basically three things you need to do during the sugar detox period. There are more to it like good exercise and removing other unhealthy diets as well. But for now these are the things you have to focus on:

1. You have to avoid eating or drinking all sugar and simple carbohydrates from your diet for 21 days, uninterrupted. There is a very long list of things you cannot eat compared to the much shorter one of recommended food. You must follow these at all times.

2. You have to watch what you eat for those three weeks. It would be recommended to keep a food journal for this task. Doing so will make it easier for you to watch out what you eat and you'll find it easier to control eating impulses. It can even encourage you to continue the food journal even after the detox period. You might also want to include a computation of your total calorie intake for each entry.

3. If you missed a day of detoxification or if you slip up and eat something you're not supposed to even just once (eating or drinking something with sugar or simple carbs), you'll have to start from zero. This will motivate you to try hurdling through the 21 days without returning to day one.

Before you do start the sugar detox process, you have to consider some of these things in your mind. But, just a warning: you have to hold steadfast. Remember what they say about beauty and health, "no pain, no gain". Not that you'll be in pain, for the most part. Here are some of the things you need to think about:

- *21 Days can feel like an eternity.*

  You may have chosen this detox plan on a whim. Maybe you just saw it in a forum or you heard someone who did well with it. Well, you'll see 21 days solidly spent on this detox is no walk in the park. It's going to be like crawling through briars in the middle of a thunderstorm. You have to keep your determination steadfast and just don't be discouraged because it will definitely prove to be a challenge. The rewards will all be worth it in the end, that's for sure.

- *You'll have to stick to it honestly.*

  Finishing your 21-day sugar detox within less than 21 days will be the easiest way to relapse into our sugar addiction. Cutting your diet plan this way will ensure the return of your problematic habit, probably more strongly than before. It is a carefully-made program that will ensure ridding both your body and your mind of the uncontrollable craving for sugar. So, just because you feel a little better after a week or two, you cannot just cut the detox process that short. It is set at 21 days for a reason.

  Absolutely don't cheat, shortcut or mess it up. If you did, even by the tiniest little bit, restart and do it properly for three weeks.

- *A one-time 3-week detox may not be enough.*

If you think a single three-week detox will work for you, don't be too sure. A lifetime worth of sugar addiction can take quite a few passes of this detox process to completely clear out. Advice: keep at it until you've been completely "cured" of the built up sugar over all those years. But do remember to take a break. Say after three weeks of uninterrupted detox, return to a normal (albeit a healthier) diet and then restart after some time following through the three weeks again.

- *It is not a lifestyle changing plan.*

It is just the tip of the ice berg, so to say. You have to decide what lifestyle you would be following after your detox. That is because you will definitely have to leave the high-carb, high-sugar lifestyle you've had before, so take a note of this. You can even use this opportunity to fix more than just your diet in your lifestyle. After all, it will be easier for you to change some of your unhealthy habits when you don't have those persistent cravings anymore. But note that this will just be a start if you want a complete lifestyle change.

- *It is adjustable to fit different individuals.*

Definitely better than most of the unchangeable diet programs, sugar detox can take form on different levels or intensity to suit your sugar use. There are some designed for those who have flat-out sugar addiction. While there is also some plans that is preferred by the ones who don't consume that much sugar, there are those that are made for slow-starters. Either that or it is because they feel that the higher level detox programs are too much. Being a bit uncomfortable with the designed plan is normal; you are trying to change your habits after all. But you should know that too much discomfort is detrimental to your progress. So, choose a detox plan that will suit your requirements.

- *The detox process pushes all the bad things out. It will let you feel in full what all that sugar was doing to your body.*

  You will definitely feel the effects of withdrawal. The worst of the effects of that built up sugar in your body will certainly show themselves during the process. Remember to keep your determination to help you overcome these things and the experiences that will obstruct the path of your detoxification in the first few days.

Your nutritionist or physician can suggest further additions to this diet as well as other things you can do to make it more effective. They can give helpful advice such as the kind of physical activity you can maintain during the detox period. If you didn't want to consult with a doctor, you can find many references on the subject. There are many discussions about tried and tested diet plans in books, articles and blogs online.

Chapter 6

Some Sugar-free Recipes

Here are some of the food products you would want to have in your diet during the sugar detox program:

- Herbs

- Vegetables (except potatoes)

- Beans

- Avocado

- Carrots

- Coconut Oil

- Eggs

- Fish

- Meat

- Nuts

- Olive Oil

- Seed-foods

- Tomatoes

- Citrus Fruits (not the sweet citrus ones though)

- Unsweetened chocolate (Dark and black chocolates are actually good for you. Even if they're quite bitter, they can substitute desserts. It is an acquired taste after all so they might take a little getting used to.)

And the stuff you need to avoid:

- Alcohol

- Flour and flour-based products

- Fried food

- Fruit juices

- Artificial sweeteners (they're worse than sugar, promise!)

- fruits

- Bread products

- Corn syrup (start checking labels, this stuff is in many things)

- Candy

- honey

- Cereal

- Maple syrup

- Cheese

- Potatoes (yes, even fries)

- Dairy products

- oatmeal

- Cream sauces

- Sugar

- Soy

- Tortillas and other corn-based crackers

- White rice

- Trans-fat (these should be in the label, look them up)

- Yogurt (even the non-fat, unsweetened ones!)

- Pasta (all of them)

- Pizza

Meatballs in Tomato Sauce

Ingredients:

- ¼ cup Parmesan cheese
- 2 lightly beaten eggs
- 1/3 cup whole wheat bread crumbs
- 12 oz. or 3 pieces sausages removed from casings
- 1 lb. ground beef (choose one with less fat)
- 1 tsp. minced garlic
- Salt
- Pepper
- Parmesan cheese for garnish

Sauce:
- 1 tbsp. minced garlic
- 2 cans tomatoes, diced and pureed
- 1 tsp. dried oregano
- 2 tsp. dried basil
- salt

Procedure:

1. Preheat the oven to 425° F. Remove the sausages and ground beef from the cold. Squeeze the sausage meat from their casings and bring both meats to room temperature.

2. Put the bread crumbs in a bowl and add 1/3 cup of hot water. Let the crumbs absorb the water before adding the garlic, salt, pepper, grated Parmesan cheese and the eggs. After mixing them well, add the meats and use your hands to combine them.

3. Prepare the pan or dish with oil or nonstick spray. Round up meatballs with your hands, using a spoon to

measure out the meat. Arrange them so they'll have space between each meatball.

4. Puree the tomatoes. After putting it in a bowl, add in the salt, herbs and garlic. Pour this sauce over the meatballs. Sprinkle the remaining cheese over them. Bake them until the sauce and the cheese is bubbling. That would take just over half an hour.

Serve it hot with more Parmesan sprinkled on the meatballs.

This recipe makes about 6 servings.

Chicken Nuggets with Almonds

Ingredients:

- 2 tbsp. olive oil
- 1 tsp. paprika
- ½ cup almond flour or almond meal
- ½ tsp. chicken seasoning
- 2 skinless chicken breasts, boneless

Procedure:

1. Preheat oven to 400° F. Prepare the pan and baking sheet with the olive oil.

2. Remove all tendons and visible fat from the chicken then cut it into nuggets (each breast piece should make about 5 pieces). Make sure they are all of the same thickness, using a kitchen mallet to even out differences.

3. Combine the rest of the ingredients in a bowl and mix well. Dip each nugget into this mixture, making sure it coats the chicken evenly. Line them up into the pan with the baking sheet.

4. Cook for around 10 minutes, until the side touching the pan is slightly browned. The nuggets become too hard and chewy when overcooked so don't overdo it. Once one side is cooked, turn the nuggets and then cook for another 10 minutes.

5. Serve hot with your favorite chicken nugget dip.

This recipe makes about 2 servings.

Muffin Pan Meal

Ingredients:

- 6 eggs
- 8 ½ oz. muffin mix (or corn bread)
- Salt
- Pepper
- 15 oz. corned beef

Procedure:

1. Grease the 12-cup muffin pan. Divide the corned beef into six of these cups. Press them down, so that it sticks to the bottom and comes up at the sides to form shells.

2. Break an egg into each shell and season with some salt and pepper.

3. Prepare muffin mix according to the instructions on the packaging. Spoon the muffin batter into the remaining 6 cups.

4. Bake at 400° F for up to 20 minutes or just when the muffins are golden brown.

5. Put the cooked egg and shell onto the muffins as toppings. Serve immediately. They could also be reheated by putting them through the microwave for a few seconds on mid-level heat.

This recipe makes 4 - 6 servings.

Chicken Skillet

Ingredients:

- 3 tbsp. olive oil
- ½ chopped green pepper
- 1 chopped onion
- 4 crushed garlic cloves
- 1 ½ lbs. boneless chicken
- Salt
- Pepper

Procedure:

1. Slice the chicken to your desired serving pieces.

2. Heat the oil in the skillet and cook the chicken until they are nearly done.

3. Add the garlic, onion and the green pepper, sauté them with the chicken.

4. You know you are finished cooking when the chicken is slightly browned and the onion has become soft.

5. After that, you can add some choice vegetables and sauté until cooked to your liking.

6. Season with salt and pepper.

Beef Barbecue Sandwiches and Burritos

Ingredients:

- Hamburger buns
- 1 packet taco seasoning
- Flour tortillas with your favorite toppings
- 1 bottle of barbecue sauce
- 5 lbs. roast beef

Procedure:

1. Shred well-cooked roast meat with a fork. Reserve half of the meat for the sandwiches. Drain any liquid left in the pot with the meat. Put the taco seasoning and stir in two cups of water with the remaining half of the meat. Cook until heated through.

2. Serve on tortillas.

3. Take the other half and stir in the barbecue sauce. Heat mixture in the microwave (or on a stove top).

4. Serve on buns.

This recipe makes about 4 servings.

Onion Rings

Ingredients:

- 2 onions, choose the white ones
- ½ red pepper powder or chili powder
- 1 tsp. ground black pepper
- Salt
- 250 ml beer
- 1 ¾ cup flour
- ¼ cup corn meal

Procedure:

1. Mix the flour and corn meal, stirring in the red and black pepper, salt and beer. Make sure all the ingredients are mixed evenly. Afterwards, cover it and let it sit for an hour.

2. In a pan, heat about 5 cm-high peanut or olive oil until it is around 370° F.

3. On a plate filled with a mound of flour, toss 5 or 6 pieces of onion rings, and then dip it in your prepared batter. Drop them one at a time into the oil.

4. Cook the rings for a few minutes until they are sufficiently browned on both sides. Drain off all oil with paper towels or by putting them on a wire rack. Salt the rings and serve hot.

This recipe makes 4-6 servings.

Eggplant Sticks

Ingredients:

- ½ cup beaten eggs
- ¾ tsp. garlic and salt powder
- 1 cup spaghetti sauce or tomato sauce of your choice
- 1 eggplant (1 ¼ lbs.)
- Seasoning of your choice

Procedure:

1. Cut eggplant into snack-sized sticks.

2. In a long bowl or on a dish, combine the garlic and salt powder, with your choice seasoning. Dip each eggplant stick into the beaten eggs then coat it in the powder mixture. Arrange them on a baking sheet.

3. Spray the laid out sticks with cooking spray. Broil the sticks for 3 minutes. Remove the baking sheet from the oven afterwards.

4. Turn the sticks and spritz them again with the cooking spray. Cook for another 2 minutes or when they are browned to your liking.

5. Serve hot. Prepare the tomato sauce as your dip.

This recipe makes about 8 servings.

Sausage Snacks

Ingredients:

- 12 oz. spicy pork sausages, ground
- 12 oz. pork sausages, ground
- Ham slices
- Scrambled eggs, fried
- mayonnaise

Procedure:

1. Preheat your broiler.

2. Mix and cook the ground pork sausage and the spicy ground pork sausage in a well-oiled skillet. Brown the ground pork over medium high heat. Drain the sausage of any liquid.

3. Process the ground pork with the mayonnaise until they are incorporated well.

4. On each ham slice, place some of the ground pork mixture and some scrambled eggs. Roll them up and secure with a toothpick.

5. Broil the rolls for 3 to 5 minutes. Check it frequently, and finishing when they are sufficiently toasted.

This recipe makes about 5-6 servings.

Roasted Chickpeas

Ingredients:

- Olive oil or cooking spray
- Salt
- 1 tsp. chili powder
- 1 tsp. paprika
- 1 tsp. coriander
- 1 tsp. cumin
- 1 tsp. garlic powder
- 1 tsp. curry powder

Procedure:

1. Preheat oven to 375° F. Drain chickpeas and let them completely dry. If you need to, you can pat dry them with a paper towel.

2. Arrange them on a baking sheet, laying them on a single layer. Roast for around half an hour, shaking the pan every ten minutes. Just make sure they don't burn. You'll know they are done when they have turned golden brown with crunchy insides instead of moist.

3. Combine all the spices in a bowl, mixing them well. Remove the chickpeas from the oven when they are done and spray them with olive oil.

4. Toss the chickpeas with the spices while they're still hot.

5. They are preferably served hot. But you can also let them cool in room temperature and then place them in airtight Ziploc bags afterwards.

This recipe makes about 3 servings.

Conclusion

Thank you again for purchasing "***Sugar Detox Guide for Beginners***: *Lose Weight Quickly, Achieve Optimal Health, Feel Energized and Eliminate Sugar Cravings Naturally*"!

I hope this book was able to help you to have a less-sugary diet and have a more positive outlook to set you up for a good and healthy lifestyle.

The next step is to create a new lifestyle that will let you live healthier and happier.

Finally, if you enjoyed this book, please take the time to share your thoughts and post a review on Amazon. It'd be greatly appreciated!

I would love for you to share your experiences, stories and encouragements with me. My email address is emmarosekindle@gmail.com

In addition, please remember to check out our Facebook page in order to find other resources and upcoming promotions:

https://www.facebook.com/joypublishing

With sincere thanks,

Emma Rose

Emma Rose

Preview Of "Paleo Desserts: Satisfy Your Sweet Tooth With Over 100 Quick and Easy Paleo Dessert Recipes and Paleo Baking Recipes"

Chapter 1

Brief History of Paleo Diet

The Sweet Effects

Why do you love sweet food? Why do you crave for more of that dessert so much? Your anatomy would tell you that sweet foods would cause the release of dopamine in the part of the brain that is associated with motivation and reward. Not only that, but studies show that sweets also produce an increased level of serotonin. Serotonin gives you that feeling of happiness and wellbeing. That's why it is better to give a box of chocolates when you want the person to be in a good mood.

Unfortunately, the quote you can't have your cake and eat it too applies here. The bad effects that sugar brings are common knowledge. The number one disease is diabetes. People are aware of diabetes and its complications. That is why even when you intensely crave for that delicious dessert, you try to control your urges and settle for nothing instead. Well, that is if your self-control is in good condition. More often than not, people would rather risk the medical condition and eat that sweet thing with all their heart.

I have had many slip ups in my own life. I went two months without chocolate...can you believe it? Then Easter came. I found that if I gave myself an inch, I would take a mile. Eating chocolate quickly got out of control. I rebelled because I was strict for so long. You may find yourself in the same situation and find it hard to balance the sugar cravings. Once the sugar cravings are there, your body craves more and then a vicious cycle begins.

Bonus Recipe:

Classic Chocolate-Strawberry Bars

This has many prehistoric ingredients but worth the effort.

Ingredients:
2 ¼ cups almond flour
½ cup coconut sugar
½ tsp baking powder
6 tbsp flaxseed meal
¼ tsp sea salt
2/3 cups arrowroot powder

6 tbsp coconut oil, melted
3 tbsp coconut milk
2 tsp vanilla extract

½ cup dark chocolate chips
½ cup fresh cut strawberries
1 tbsp fresh lemon juice
Handful chopped almonds (optional)

Procedure:
Preheat the oven to 350°F. Combine in a bowl 2 ¼ cups almond flour, ½ cup coconut sugar, ½ teaspoon baking powder, 6 tablespoons flaxseed meal, ¼ teaspoon sea salt and 2/3 cups arrowroot powder. In a separate bowl, whisk the following: 6 tablespoons melted coconut oil, 3 tablespoons coconut milk and 2 teaspoons vanilla extract. Mix together the wet and dry ingredients using a gloved hand. This will form soft dough. Take note not to over mix this.

Reserve ½ cup of dough to be used later. Place the remaining dough on an 8" x 8" baking pan lined with parchment paper. Top with ½ cup dark chocolate chips. Cover the chips with fresh cut strawberries. Drizzle with 1 tablespoon fresh lemon juice and then drizzle with the extra dough plus an extra handful of almonds. Bake the dough for 20 minutes then lower the heat to 325°F and then bake for another 10 minutes. It should turn into a beautiful golden color crumble bar. Cut and serve.

Check out the rest of "Paleo Desserts: Satisfy Your Sweet Tooth With Over 100 Quick and Easy Paleo Dessert Recipes and Paleo Baking Recipes" on Amazon.

Or go to: http://amzn.to/1lZNcVI

Check Out My Other Books

Below you'll find some of my other books also available on Amazon and Kindle. Search for these titles on the Amazon website to find them.

Paleo Free Diet Guide for Beginners: Over 50 Paleo Free Recipes for Optimal Health & Fast Weight Loss

Paleo Desserts: Satisfy Your Sweet Tooth With Over 100 Quick & Easy Paleo Dessert Recipes & Paleo Baking Recipes

Raw Food Diet Guide: Lose Weight Quickly, Achieve Optimal Health & Feel Energized with the Raw Food Diet & Raw Food Recipes

Clean Eating Guide: Lose Weight Quickly, Achieve Optimal Health & Feel Energized with Clean Eating For Busy Families & Clean Eating Recipes

Alkaline Diet Guide: Lose Weight Quickly, Achieve Optimal Health & Feel Energized with the Alkaline Diet & Alkaline Recipes

Coconut Flour Recipes for Optimal Health & Quick Weight Loss: Gluten Free Recipes for Celiac Disease, Gluten Sensitivities & Paleo Free Diets

Almond Flour Recipes for Optimal Health & Quick Weight Loss: Gluten Free Recipes for Celiac Disease, Gluten Sensitivities & Paleo Free Diets

Wheat Free Diet for Beginners: Lose Weight Quickly, Achieve Optimal Health & Feel Energized with Gluten Free Recipes for Celiac Disease, Gluten Sensitivities & Paleo Free Diets

Detox Diet Guide: Lose Weight Quickly, Achieve Optimal Health & Feel Energized Through the 10 Day Detox

Sugar Detox Guide for Beginners: Lose Weight Quickly, Achieve Optimal Health, Feel Energized & Eliminate Sugar Cravings Naturally

Ketogenic Diet Guide for Beginners: How to Achieve Rapid Weight Loss, Optimal Health & Unstoppable Energy with Ketogenic Diet Recipes

Anti Inflammatory Diet for Beginners: Lose Weight Fast, Optimize Health, Slow Aging, Fight Inflammation, Conquer Pain & Increase Energy with the Anti Inflammation Diet Recipes

One Last Thing...

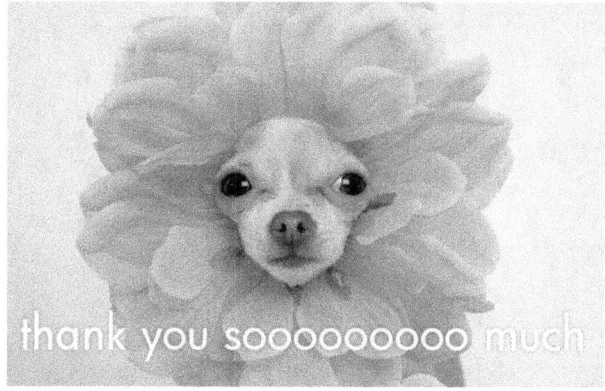

thank you soooooooooo much

If you believe that this book is worth sharing, would you please take the time to let others know how it affected your life? If it turns out to make a difference in the lives of others, they will be forever grateful to you, as will I.

www.ingramcontent.com/pod-product-compliance
Lightning Source LLC
Chambersburg PA
CBHW060109300526
45791CB00018B/954